HOW TO HAVE A HEALTHY MARRIED SEX LIFE

7 key secrets to a successful marriage

Brittany Valentine

Table Of Contents

Introduction

Sexual recurrence in marriage can change over the long haul, yet sex doesn't need to get exhausting in a drawn-out relationship. As the years go by and you age, your connection ought to improve. Sex with your accomplice can turn out to be more fulfilling because you know one another's preferences, aversions, propensities, and inclinations.

Keeping a solid sexual coexistence is difficult. Couples get into an everyday practice and life gets going. Add kids and requesting positions to the situation, and keeping up with any kind of closeness is an overwhelming errand. Be that as it may, notwithstanding how hard it very well may be, it's significant. Great sex keeps couples associated. Fortunately, there are attempted and tried tips and procedures to assist with keeping that flash alive.

Keeping awake until late looking over web-based entertainment to stay away from closeness with your accomplice or, more regrettably, professing to be snoozing, isn't great for your marriage. In any case, on the off chance that you wind up staying away from sex, you're in good company: Roughly one lady in 10 encounters a diminishing in her sex drive eventually in her life.

"That plunge can occur for various reasons, including the normal movement of your relationship over the long run," However you shouldn't abandon having an extraordinary sexual coexistence whenever you're hitched. Closeness is vital to having a solid, utilitarian, and by and large blissful relationship."

Sex is an oxygen-consuming movement, and that implies it can help your heart's well-being. "One vivacious demonstration of intercourse consumes 180 calories - which, in all honesty, is identical to around 20 minutes of delicate running or playing a 9-opening round of golf."

Getting playful with your soul mate can likewise help your state of mind. Sex discharges endorphins, your cerebrum's "vibe great" synthetics. Also, the chemicals delivered during sex might bring down gloom and uneasiness levels and lift invulnerability. Having customary intercourse with your accomplice can likewise further develop rest, upgrade life span, and safeguard cerebrum capability.

Sexuality : A Gift From God

As Modern Holy people, we comprehend that sexuality is a gift from God. We likewise comprehend that our bodies are not obstructions to our otherworldliness; rather they are vehicles toward it. We accept that our epitome works with our capacity to turn out to be more similar to God.

The integrity is not set in stone by how we manage this gift. We can utilize our sexuality to elevate or belittle. Figuring out how to cherish and be adored through the body is central to our otherworldly and social limit and permits us to encounter something of godliness through such significant love. It is additionally basic to joy in marriage. While many naturally dread delight, actually God needs this for us with regards to marriage since it is a gift to us, since it supports us, and on the grounds that God believes us should have satisfaction.

To work on seeing sexuality as a present, give yourself full consent to find and get joy. This is particularly significant for ladies who have realized time and again that ongoing discipline is an uprightness. To allow oneself to be supported physically is a profound graciousness to oneself as well regarding a companion.

Sexuality is a gift to all kinds of people. God has prepared the two sexual orientations similarly, yet in an unexpected way, for closeness and joy. Yet, many dishonestly discover that sexuality is basic to men's prosperity yet not to ladies'. A few ladies view their restricted craving as a statement of womanliness and accept that being a decent spouse requires dealing with the husband's sexual necessities. Of course, a spouse's uninvolved convenience of a husband's longings rapidly transforms her underlying interest into disdain. Feeling committed to engage in sexual relations will constantly kill energy. It further leaves the two accomplices feeling undesired, misjudged, and disliked.

Couples ought to believe solid sexual satisfaction to be an objective to deal with together, and they ought to perceive that the cycle will require some investment. Recently wedded couples come to the relationship with a wide range of inclinations toward sex. Some may be good to go and agreeable to their sexuality, while others might be oblivious, have discovered that examining sex is not, or perhaps assimilated the thought that sexuality is risky and an expected danger to otherworldliness and steadiness in a couple. It might require investment for one or two accomplices to manage these sorts of sentiments, so persistence and openness are of the utmost importance for this cycle.

Having persistence might imply that a recent several don't become engrossed with quickly fulfilling their marriage but rather center around shared investigation and joy, especially from the get-go. Since ladies ordinarily stimulate more leisurely than men, it is important not to rush towards intercourse. Intercourse on the wedding night frequently leaves unpracticed spouses inadequately stimulated. Also, when excitement is low (as will be the situation when tension is high), ladies might encounter torment, which need not be the situation. Beginning agony will cause expanded uneasiness and lower excitement the following time, perhaps prompting more torment and in the end sexual aversion.3 Beginning gradually and fostering a strong association through exotic ways of behaving is substantially more critical to the drawn-out government assistance of the couple than fulfilling rapidly once wedded.

See your ability to typify love as an expertise you can create
It is essential to see sexual closeness as a language through which one can cherish and be adored, want, and be wanted. It is a language you can turn out to be more conversant in with training and consideration. For instance, you can utilize contact to impart dismissal or qualification, or you can utilize contact to convey love, want, and appreciation. Consider what you as of now discuss in your cozy commitment with your life partner. What does your companion comprehend about you in the manner you contact? What do you communicate about how you feel about your companion? What could you change in the messages you offer through your actual commitment?

Offering acknowledgment and benevolence through sexuality is an expertise you can create. In this light, want isn't something that happens to you in marriage. Want is, all things considered, an outflow of picking your mate — deciding to focus on and care for themselves and offer your sexuality with them. This sort of significance presented through cozy contact makes sex a bringing together and securing experience and what makes sex alluring for blissful couples.That is trailed by the stage in which many couples start a family. Having youngsters fundamentally changes a couple's closeness. "It's normal for a couple's sexual coexistence to decline in the wake of having a child in view of the weariness and absence of private time,". "Be that as it may, many couples' sexual experiences don't recuperate after they escape the child zone. Needs shift to bringing up children and shuffling professions and family obligations."

Regardless of whether you have kids, the novelty of the relationship wears off following three or four years together. Normally, this is when sex turns out to be more everyday practice. "Closeness separates at this stage since couples don't discuss their sexual coexistence,"

Sexual Barriers

Other than the development of a relationship, different variables can prompt less closeness, as well. Profession and family tensions can gobble up your time and zap your energy. Social damages or feelings of disdain can foster over the long haul. One of the most widely recognized? Feeling overpowered and angry that your accomplice isn't assisting however much you would like.

On the off chance that your accomplice won't resolve these issues, they will keep on influencing your relationship and sexuality, and observe that this is a cognizant choice on their part not to fill here. If so and your accomplice decides not to develop, yet their decision is affecting you and your relationship, you should look for advice. Certain individuals, ordinarily, need to develop and change. Others dread development and change, so they can oppose looking for help, even in regions where such development would work on all aspects of their lives.

That is while having a heart-to-heart can help. "Put your accomplice down and say, 'Look, this it resembles to be a lady with these children in my day to day existence at the present time and with my profession. Do you get it? Might you at any point back up and help me?" "You truly need to discuss it on the grounds that the disdain that develops around sensations of disparity is one of the greatest enemies of closeness and sexuality."

As well as examining relationship concerns, it's fundamental to have discussions about your sexual coexistence, as well, regardless of whether it's troublesome or abnormal from the get go. Simply start the discussion by posing inquiries like:

What are a few sexual exercises we've done that you are truly delighted in?
How are a few things you'd like to attempt?
Is there anything you might want to accomplish pretty much?
How associated with me are you feeling recently?
Increment Closeness
It's essential to focus on how you and your accomplice are connecting with each other all through the room.

Closeness will in general follow an example as a relationship develops. Couples recently enamored commonly experience sensations of closeness and fervor and have normal sex.

That is trailed by the stage in which many couples start a family. Having kids fundamentally changes a couple's closeness. "It's normal for a couple's sexual coexistence to decline in the wake of having a child due to the depletion and absence of private time,". "Yet, many couples' sexual experiences don't recuperate after they escape the child zone. Needs shift to bringing up children and shuffling professions and family obligations."

Regardless of whether you have kids, the freshness of the relationship wears off following three or four years together. Ordinarily, this is when sex turns out to be a more daily schedule. "Closeness separates at this stage since couples don't discuss their sexual coexistence,"

Recognize Your Necessities

Recognize what causes you to want to have intercourse. In contrast to men — who are effectively excited — ladies' longing is a more progressive cycle. "As a rule, ladies' longing begins with an association with their own sexuality or their accomplice of some sort or another. Most ladies frequently should be loose, not stressed over their plan for the day, and feeling an association with their accomplice to make way for sexual closeness,".

To get in that frame of mind, ponder what causes you to feel loose and erotic. Perhaps it's kissing or contacting or talking personally with your accomplice. It may very well be a glass of wine, a pleasant supper or giggling together. Whenever you've pinpointed what causes you to feel prepared for sexual closeness, share that data with your companion so you can cooperate to get those things going.

Grasping your accomplice's assumptions, wants, likes, and aversions is significant — not just as far as their sexual style and solace level, however what they need to feel cherished and appreciated, and at last more joyful in your relationship.

We as a whole express and feel love diversely — or have an alternate "way to express affection" — and understanding those distinctions can assume a major part in keeping up with closeness in your marriage.

Solid sexuality in marriage ends up being clear when the two accomplices can communicate their sexual longings and necessities to their accomplice. It is a characteristic of solace and a sound correspondence design.

By communicating what you want to improve for your sexual fulfillment, you can direct your accomplice about what you genuinely need. It can work on your sexual comprehension of one another, rather than permitting presumptions to lead you off course.

Have Transparent Correspondence

On the off chance that you're not speaking with your accomplice, how might they understand what fulfills you? Thus, how might you comprehend what they appreciate and what stimulates them?

Not an incident couples who have the most fulfilling sex lives are likewise the people who impart uninhibitedly and transparently. Working it out with your accomplice is critical to making a shared grasping that prompts closeness… which thusly can prompt extraordinary sex.

"Again and again, ladies say 'I'm somewhat drained,' 'I want to shower,' or 'It's anything but a great time.' However the couples who really try to have intercourse consistently — regardless of whether it's not the ideal situation — have seriously fulfilling sex lives,". In the event that your accomplice starts a sexual experience, take a stab at obliging it to see where it leads you. "Numerous ladies report feeling excitement after the closeness has started," he adds. Obviously, on the off chance that it doesn't get you in that frame of mind, you ought to constantly feel qualified to stop.

Open correspondence is the foundation of any sound and flourishing relationship, be it heartfelt, kinship, or expert. It is a two-way course of trading data, thoughts, and sentiments among people, and it assumes an essential part in building trust, understanding, and shared regard.

One of the main advantages of open correspondence is that it cultivates a feeling of genuineness and straightforwardness between people. At the point when the two players feel open to sharing their contemplations and feelings unafraid of judgment or repercussion, it establishes a protected and steady climate for development and improvement. This permits people to communicate their requirements, wants, and concerns openly, prompting a superior comprehension of one another's viewpoint and necessities.

Open correspondence additionally advances undivided attention and sympathy, which are basic abilities in any relationship. By effectively paying attention to each other, people can acquire a more profound comprehension of their accomplice's contemplations and sentiments. This aids in settling clashes as well as fortifies the connection between people, as it shows a readiness to help and approve each other's feelings.

Two primary sorts of correspondence that lead to expanded sexual fulfillment are verbal and non-verbal sexual correspondence. Does talking or non-verbally inferring about sex lead to more prominent sexual fulfillment? That might be some unacceptable inquiry.

Scientists have archived that the sort of correspondence used isn't what's generally significant. Whether a couple is content with the kind of sex correspondence makes the biggest difference. Think about imparting sexual inclinations: examine sexual preferences, aversions, wants, and sexual recurrence.

While examining inclinations, various discussions about sex in marriage could surface. In some cases couples talk about their inclinations, however different times couples examine sexual errors or issues. These discussions about sex in marriage can be pivotal for couples to comprehend the other and ought not be dreaded. As couples convey, they can comprehend what their life partner needs in the room and better take care of sexual cravings.

Correspondence is the way into a sound and dynamic sexual coexistence in a conjugal relationship, so talk with each other more. Talking about shallow things can be fun, yet make sure to go further to lay out closeness, as a matter of fact.

Share your deepest considerations and sentiments with each other routinely. Sexual closeness is a proceeding with interaction of discovery. Genuine closeness through correspondence is something that can make sex perfect.

It's not difficult to set sex aside for later when you're in a constant phase of life. However, the main way you will keep a close association with your accomplice is by focusing on it. "Couples who timetable the chance to associate with one another have better, more joyful connections," says Kraft. "It doesn't need to bring about sex like clockwork. It's more about making time to have some good times together."

Get a sitter and timetable a night out, or just put the children to sleep early so you can have some alone time. Have some time off from your insane plan for getting work done to meet each other for lunch, or step away from your home redesign task and remain for the time being at a lodging. Sort out ways you can set aside a few minutes for one another.

The world puts a great deal of expectations on your time. Whether it's rearranging kids to the everyday schedule for that significant show to the board, shuffling family, vocation and different stressors can overpower. Therefore, you might feel you lack the capacity to deal with sex.

That is the reason working sex into your schedule is considerably more significant. Recollect that sex doesn't necessarily need to be unconstrained. While many might recoil that booking sex isn't heartfelt, it gives a valuable chance to lay out more prominent closeness with your accomplice.

In the event that you and your accomplice both have occupied plans, put down a point in time during the week for a night out to keep up with your recurrence of sex. Change up your action and stay present at the time to take out interruptions and keep your relationship from entering a trench.

"Getting some down time to enjoy with your accomplice is quite possibly the most cherishing thing you can accomplish for one another,". "I recommend that couples get a duplicate of the book 8 Sexual Evenings, which offers eight exotic exercises that will tell you and your accomplice the best way to satisfy one another." Alternate choosing an action and you'll associate all the more energetically with your accomplice.

Feel Attractive

There's no question that feeling attractive can help your charisma. So you should invest energy doing the things that cause you to feel exotic, whether that is wearing provocative outfits or underwear, perusing romance books or erotica, or getting bendy at yoga class. The point is to zero in on your necessities.

So how would you feel provocative and meriting love? One of the quickest ways of working on your relationship with your body generally speaking is to pay attention to it. The most vital phase in your course of reconnecting with your body is permitting yourself to pay attention to the message it needs to tell you.

Setting the mind-set for sex in marriage can prompt expanded sexual fulfillment, excitement, and enthusiasm. Send a hot message to your companion during the day. Additionally, get some margin for foreplay like sluggish, delicate kissing that could prompt profound kissing that can assist with elevating sexual excitement and enthusiasm. Requiring an end of the week escape to a lodge or inn can give adequate couple alone time — like a wedding trip. As you set the state of mind for sexual enthusiasm, joy and fulfillment can have large amounts of your marriage.

"We have a wonderful sexual coexistence, "Most likely on the grounds that I'm never at any point sloppy at home. I generally wear little slips and charming artful dance shoes in the house. I give my very best to feel provocative — it keeps the zest in our marriage. I could never hang out at home in warm up pants. The sex never disappears for us. We have great actual science, despite the fact that there are days that I need to kill him."

Reclassify Closeness

Closeness in a relationship is a sensation of being close, and genuinely associated and upheld. It implies having the option to share an entire scope of contemplations, sentiments and encounters that we have as people. It includes being open and talking through your viewpoints and feelings, letting your gatekeeper down (being powerless), and showing another person how you feel and what your deepest desires are.

Closeness is developed after some time, and it requires persistence and exertion from the two accomplices to make and keep up with. Finding closeness with somebody you love can be one of the most remunerating parts of a relationship.

Aside from profound and sexual closeness, you can likewise be personal mentally, casually, monetarily, profoundly, imaginatively (for instance, remodeling your home) and on occasion of emergency (functioning collectively during difficult stretches).

"Individuals frequently think sex must be a major creation with intercourse and climaxes. At the point when in all actuality, what's generally vital to couples, particularly to numerous ladies, is to associate and be close. Being close can be essentially as straightforward as talking and nestling or tenderly contacting,"

Request that your accomplice center around "outercourse": contacting, rubbing, kissing and nestling. Also, examine the chance of having these kinds of meetings without feeling committed to engage in sexual relations.

"The most compelling thing is to make having a personal association with your accomplice a need," Contemplate what causes you to feel close and what you appreciate physically. And afterward ask yourself how you can make that with your accomplice."

Who says you need to trust that your significant other will start sex? Rather than hanging tight for him to drop indicates that he needs to have intercourse this evening, you can decide to take the principal action. Settle on the decision telling your better half you have made some arrangements for him this evening. Or on the other hand maneuver him into the room and disrobe him, letting him know what you believe he should do straightaway.

Assuming responsibility will assist with touching off your sexual coexistence in marriage and pay off no doubt. At the point when he is accustomed to starting sex, your better half will presumably find you assuming responsibility for your sexual coexistence invigorating. Try not to be modest! At the point when you assume command, you get to pick when, where, and how, permitting you the chance to pick what works for yourself as well as your body. Keep in mind, when you assume responsibility, pick sex places that let you assume command over the activity.

Toward the start of a relationship, couples appreciate profound, hot kissing, and they contact each other in exciting ways. In any case, as a relationship develops, that affectionate way of behaving can assume a lower priority in relation to errands and unremarkable exercises. Channel your inward teen and kiss, embrace, and cuddle your accomplice as you did when you initially met. Doing so will assist with keeping your marriage physically alive.

Look for Help When Required

In the event that you and your accomplice are experiencing difficulty fabricating and keeping a satisfying sexual coexistence, you might have to look for help from a prepared proficient person who can assist you with doing whatever it may take to determine the issue.

Converse with a specialist. In the event that clinical issues like erectile brokenness (ED) or vaginal dryness are obstructing your sexual coexistence, a clinical expert can endorse suitable treatment.

Look for mentoring: Marriage mentoring (additionally called couples treatment) can be exceptionally compelling for opening the lines of correspondence among you and your life partner and sorting out techniques for further developing sex and closeness.

Connect with a sex specialist. Sex treatment is a type of talk treatment, not involved treatment, that is utilized to assist people and couples with resolving sexual issues.

Working with a sex specialist, alone or together, can assist you with investigating any close to home or relationship that may be influencing your sexual coexistence.

Conclusion

Hitched sex doesn't need to be exhausting, despite the fact that it periodically is. It's likewise been displayed to have a large group of different benefits, for example, brought down circulatory strain, less pressure, more prominent closeness, and, surprisingly, a diminished separation rate.

Review that during a marriage, there will definitely be highs and lows in how much sex. Sexual recurrence can be affected by a few variables, including youngsters, stress, and sickness. Fortunately there are heaps of techniques to pick things back up and zest things up in the event that your sexual life has run into a difficult situation.

Is it safe to say that you are in a physically sound relationship? You and your accomplice will interface all the more profoundly assuming you approach them with deference, share your fantasies, and timetable incessant sex registrations. Hitched couples will have a solid sexual life because of these connections and sex exhortation.